HOW THE BRCA2 GENE

IMPACTED MY LIFE

MARY ELLEN DREHER

HOW THE BRCA2 GENE

IMPACTED MY LIFE

MARY ELLEN DREHER

TABLE OF CONTENTS

CHAPTER 1

TAPESTRY STUDY

We invite you to participate in the Tapestry study, whose goal it is to understand how patient care may be impacted when results from DNA sequencing are in the medical record," states the message that appears with my downloading e-mail. "The Tapestry study is a screening test. It looks at 11 genes associated with BRCA-related hereditary breast and ovarian cancer, Lynch syndrome and familial hypercholesterolemia. It is not a diagnostic test, nor does it look at all of the genes associated with hereditary ovarian cancer," continues the dialogue.

Hmmmm…. My attention has been captured. *Should I consider a genetic study or is this a really bad idea? I did have ovarian cancer when I was 38 years old. But that was 25 years ago, and nothing has happened since. I am pretty sure I don't have any genetic mutations for cancer. I have no family history of breast or ovarian cancer. But still . . . I do have a daughter who has become concerned here lately as to her risk of ovarian cancer. If all this testing were to come back negative, it would provide her with peace of mind.*

Three days later on October 23, 2020, I respond to the e-mail and join Mayo Clinic's Health Tapestry Genomic Sequencing in Clinical Practice study. I am sent a kit into which I am to collect a specific amount of sputum. I spit into the collection container and mail it off to the lab in the pre-addressed box. Then I wait. The information given to me was that the test results would take up to twelve weeks to be reported. That was simple.

Several months go by and I do receive the fun results for the ancestry and genetic traits part of the study. I am 95% of European ancestry with 5% of Middle Eastern and African heritage. Mixed in there is a 0.8% Ashkenazi Jewish. I find out later this is important as 2% of those of Ashkenazi Jewish descent have a BRCA mutation. The results say I am not lactose intolerant (knew that). I have not adapted to be able to avoid malaria (Oh really!). I do not have the adaptation to be able to thrive in lower-oxygen environments at high altitudes (guess I'll stay on the plains). I do have a genotype associated with the ability to adapt in cold climates (Brr… doesn't seem like it some days in this cold MN climate). Along with lots of other useless tidbits, I learn I have brown eyes, tend towards curly hair, am taller, and tend to tan rather than sunburn; all things I have somehow managed to figure out after being on earth for 63 years. But what I really want to know, do I have a gene coding for cancer, is suspended in the health results that only say, "pending." I think this is very strange.

Towards the end of January 2021, my husband is also invited to join this same study. He signs up on February 2, 2021, and submits his saliva sample a few days later. Ten weeks later, on April 19, 2021, his results are flashed to us as "ready." He is negative for all eleven of the genes they are testing for that code for cancer. Hurrah, at least our daughter has a fighting chance!

Puzzled as to why he has received his results and I have not, I send an e-mail to Helix, the company being used by Mayo for this study, "I signed up for the Helix genetic study back in October 2020. The information originally stated that we would receive results by twelve weeks. It has now been five months and there are still no medical results. I did get the basic genetic characteristics results, but I am just curious why I still haven't gotten my medical results…?" Helix does promptly respond, "Our systems indicate that your sequencing has been sent out for interpretation. At this time, I cannot give you a time frame … Your Health results are taking longer to sequence than previously stated. We are unfortunately backlogged due to Covid 19." I find this all very confusing. Yes, maybe Covid is slowing down their results but that doesn't explain how someone who signed up after me has already received their results and I haven't. I am convinced that they have lost my sample and/or my results and are finding it convenient to blame it on Covid. It doesn't occur to me until later that they are simply not telling me the truth; that they do know the results and because they are positive, they are not ready to tell me. If I could read between the lines, it would say, "Your results were positive. Therefore, we sent them to be confirmed by a second company."

Three more months go by. I send several more e-mails to this company and each time I am told that my results, "are delayed due to supply chain issues" or "covid testing taking priority." Finally, on July 26, they report that "it looks like your results are in a recent batch that should be released by Helix any day now." Coincidently, Mayo sends an email three days later that says "you will receive an email from Helix very soon, with instructions on how to access your results on the Helix website. <u>As a participant in this study, a Mayo Clinic genetic counselor would like to review your results with you over the phone</u>." This should have been my clue that Mayo has already known the results for some time, and they are not good. Afterall, they never requested to talk to my hubby by phone to discuss his results.

It isn't until July 31, 2021, nine months after signing up for this study that I get the results. "You were found to have an actionable* variant in the BRCA2 gene that is associated with a genetic condition called Hereditary Breast and Ovarian Cancer (HBOC). Individuals with HBOC have an increased risk for certain types of cancer, including breast, ovarian, prostate, and others."

A numbness spreads over me. *Why did I think joining this study was a good idea? I would have been better off never knowing. What I had hoped would provide peace of mind to my daughter has opened a yawning pit of anguish and anxiety.*

CHAPTER 2

THE PLAN FOR BRCA2 POSITIVE

ME

am now 63 years old and have lived 25 years without any cancer reoccurrence. I have no desire to make any "might be possible cancer" a focus of my life. I can't live that way. But the question remains, should I ignore what was better unknown or try to pursue some interventions, some of which are of a huge magnitude in order to attempt to prevent what might happen? The medical community seems to be in a huge rush now to push me down this path towards interventions. No one seemed to care much before, and my cancer diagnosis 25 years ago has pretty much been forgotten. When I think about it later, the whole process of the genetic testing makes me angry. Helix and Mayo have known for at least six months but kept trying to pretend they didn't by blaming other issues and now, it is all a big rush for me to respond.

I take a breath and step back. There is no emergency here. I don't have cancer. The first intervention I request is to be retested by another reputable company to make sure this is an accurate result and can be used to drive any decisions made going forward and will be accepted by health insurance companies. After being led along for nine months, I do not trust the results I am being given. And it is not the first time such a test result has been wrong. I decide to give a blood sample this time as it has a higher rate of reliability than saliva and proceed to do so in early August. But if I was hoping for a different result, I will be disappointed. This test confirms the original finding of a "pathogenic variant (mutation) in the BRCA2 gene associated with Hereditary Breast and Ovarian Cancer syndrome."

So what is the big deal with this genetic mutation and what are its implications? BRCA1 and BRCA2 genes code for proteins that work to suppress cancer cells, mostly in breast tissue, and help to repair any DNA damage that occurs in the course of normal life. If they are missing or damaged, the cells cannot repair themselves and they go on to grow unchecked and become cancerous. BRCA2 is found on chromosome 13 while BRCA1 is found on chromosome 17 so they have slightly different cancer type expressions when missing. BRCA2 is associated with a 45 -83% lifetime risk, according to Mayo genetics, of developing breast cancer by age 70 (the average risk for the general population is 12%), a 27% risk of developing ovarian cancer by age 80 (the general population has a 1-2% risk). I think I have that one covered already. BRCA2 mutations also are associated with a higher risk of pancreatic cancers and melanoma than the general population.

Well, if that isn't all depressing. And how is one even supposed to begin to deal with statistics like that? My first reaction is to have a double mastectomy without reconstruction and get it over with. I don't want to be thinking about breast cancer every moment for the rest of my life. But after doing significant research on double mastectomies, I realize that they are not benign surgeries either. Many women have chronic pain afterward. Others have numbness and upper body muscle weakness. I am a fairly healthy 64-year-old by now. I operate a chainsaw. I lift weights. I'm active. I do not want a life where I am cancer free but simply existing because I am debilitated and in pain constantly. And finally, having my breasts removed will remove any chance of having a meaningful intimate relationship with my husband. I am distressed to say the least about the dismal statistics but can't decide what I want to do.

In October, I meet with a doctor from the breast clinic at Mayo. We go through my options: 1. Do nothing (that is not encouraged at all) 2. Have a double mastectomy (see reservations above) 3. Start taking aromatase inhibitors to help prevent cancer and/or 4. Monitor with alternating mammograms and breast MRIs every six months. I groan at each of them. I hate visiting medical facilities and doctors and have no desire to visit there constantly. Taking aromatase inhibitors sounds interesting but it is mostly a "hit and miss, maybe" approach. No one knows if I will actually get the kind of cancer that is prevented by drugs that block estrogen production and uptake. So there is a chance that I'm taking a toxic drug that is providing no benefit to me personally. I lean heavily away from their use after I read the side effects: hot flashes, night sweats, join pain by 50% of those taking it, muscle pain, and bone loss. I am back to the same issues of decreased quality of life to treat what currently doesn't exist. I don't know what to do.

Before I leave my breast appointment, I am offered the opportunity to join another study, "GENetic Risk Estimation of Breast Cancer Prior to decisions on preventative therapy uptake, risk reduction surgery, or intensive imaging surveillance: A study to determine if a polygenic risk score influences the decision-making options among high-risk women." The polygenic risk score will take into account genetic risk factors, known as single nucleotide polymorphisms (SNPs) for breast cancer. While individually, these SNP risk factors are of little clinical value, when combined as a polygenic risk score (PRS), they yield a strong risk factor for breast cancer and can be used to personalize breast cancer risk. In other words, the polygenic risk score is an analyzing of 30 or more genes that influence whether a person develops cancer and coming up with a projection for any one particular person as to what their personal chances are of developing breast cancer. At first, I reject the idea of joining another study. I am already overwhelmed by all the information and decisions being thrown at me but the more I think about it, I wonder if it could provide me with the information to make a definitive choice as to the direction I should go. And so I sign up for one more genetic study. While I wait for the results, I try to go about life as normally as possible.

This time, I do not have as long to wait. Within eight weeks, the results are back. "I have good news," are the first words from the doctor's mouth when I sit down with her. "You are in the lowest 7th percentile on the polygenic risk scoring. Because you had a hysterectomy at age 38," she says, "I assess that you have a 9% risk of developing breast cancer in 5 years, an 18% risk in 10 years, and a lifetime risk of 27%." That figure is still high compared to the general population, but I now know which direction I am going. At least for the present time, I will alternate the mammogram and breast MRI every six months. If any abnormality ever shows up, I will opt immediately for a double mastectomy without reconstruction. Now that I have made this decision, we have to come up with a plan for safely performing the MRI as I am allergic to the gadolinium dye that they use. This will be my biggest roadblock to following through on this decision.

CHAPTER 3

PATH OF INTENSIVE MONITORING

In November of 2021, after loading up on methylprednisolone and Zyrtec, an antihistamine, I successfully traverse the breast MRI. All findings are negative. I can breathe a sigh of relief, at least for six months. I begin to move on with life and focus on the future. And then, "your Cologuard test is positive." Is there no end to this craziness? Is this what old age is all about? Waiting for the cancer shoe to drop? I reject that premise. I choose to live my life in freedom from such fear, God willing – to treasure each day for what it is.

Another six months goes by, and my regular mammogram is scheduled for May of 2022. I have no more than gotten home for a few hours and I make the call back to see if more imaging is needed. "Yes," says the voice, "you need to call to set up a time for more imaging." *You have got to be kidding me.* I return the next day to the clinic for diagnostic imaging of my right breast where they can't quite make out what they are seeing. Afterall, I have dense breasts which makes for challenging imaging anyway. I am not at all in the mood for this. My breasts tend to be sore on a good day without someone putting them in a vise. Now for the diagnostic imaging, a 6x6" plate or even smaller is used to depress that area of breast tissue even further. I grit my teeth and make it through the first round the best that I can. Then I am asked to wait until someone checks the images in case they need some more. Pretty soon, the tech is back again for more. I grit my teeth again and sob my way through the next round of torture. I am about to totally lose any emotional control that I might have had. Whoever said that mammograms are only "pressure" and not pain do not know what they are talking about. All I want to do is get as far away from this place as possible. I mentally make the decision that if the tech comes back the third time, I am going to get up and walk out.

"You can go," Finally is sent my way.

The images are read as normal, and I am able to push this trauma out of my mind for another six months. I diligently set up for the yearly breast MRI in December. I ask my primary doctor for the pre-medication orders of methylprednisolone and Zyrtec to try to prevent the allergic reaction I had previously experienced. She insists that the protocol is for methylprednisolone and Benadryl, the standard antihistamine. I try to explain to her that this is not what I used the prior time or what worked. Finally, I give in and agree to try the meds stipulated by the protocol.

The day of the MRI, I do my pre-meds as ordered and proceed through the procedure with no immediate reaction. *Well that is done!* I breathe a sigh of relief. I am done for another six months or so I think. But as I undress for bed a couple of hours later, I show my husband the red raised rash and hives developing on my arms and legs. They are just beginning to itch. This will go on for several days. *So much for the pre-medication working to prevent this.*

And then one day later, I read the MRI report. "Interval development of a curvilinear nodular non-mass enhancement in the subareolar right breast, slightly lateral, slightly inferior anterior depth. Differential considerations include an intraductal process such as papillomas or possibly inflamed periductal fibrosis; however, atypia or malignancy cannot be entirely excluded." *Why would I think that I would be home free?* It has been nothing but agony since I agreed to this path of aggressive monitoring for cancer. And of course, the recommendation is for a right diagnostic mammogram and a second look ultrasound examination of the right breast finding. If there are no correlating mammographic or ultrasound findings, MRI guided biopsy is recommended. I am in a panic. I can't tolerate another breast smashing mammogram. Is there no way to escape this lunacy? I ask, if it is going to end in another MRI anyway, if I can just do the MRI in spite of the allergy and get it over with in one fell swoop?

"Oh no," is the response, "we can't do that without doing the other tests first." Totally frustrated at the lack of flexibility of all involved, I finally give in to all the pressure to follow the protocol and schedule the diagnostic mammogram and ultrasound. The mammogram shows nothing, but the ultrasound is able to see the area identified by the MRI. "It looks like inflamed periductal fibrosis," says the radiologist who checks the results. "I don't think it is cancer. You can have a biopsy now or wait another six months and see if anything develops further. But I don't think you need to worry too much." I am relieved. But in the radiologist recommendations, he writes, "recommend an MRI guided biopsy." Really? So we are right back to doing the test I am allergic to with no real reason to do so at this moment. Didn't I offer to do this before we wasted money on the mammogram and the US? But no, that just was not possible.

And my breast clinic doctor, whom I have asked to see for her opinion, now gloms onto the recommendation and can't let it go. If I have to do another reaction producing MRI, I wonder if I can wait the six months until June, have the MRI and do the biopsy at that time if necessary to limit my exposure to the dye. But again, the answer is "No, we can't do that?" I feel unsupported, unheard, and am left swimming with no acceptable options. I remind her that our original plan was to move forward with the bilateral mastectomies if anything was ever found. "Can I see a surgeon?" I finally implore, "Mastectomies would solve the need for all these tests."

With resolve that this is the right path, I show up at the surgeon's office a few weeks later for a consultation. He sits down and addresses my hubby and I, "The statistics show that for a woman your age, intensive monitoring and other interventions we have these days will result in your life expectancy being just as great as if you have the mastectomies. Mastectomies will result in your being numb, can result in infections, and you might not like the cosmetic result. There is no statistical benefit to having mastectomies. If it is the MRI allergy that is your primary concern, there is molecular breast imaging and contrast enhanced mammograms for screening." Nothing like dumping a bucket of cold water on one's head. I just stare at him over the top of my suffocating mask.

"You look skeptical?" he questions. I don't know what to say. I think there is something missing in this research, something this young surgeon is not acknowledging. What I am hearing is that the end point of the research was length of life. The studies have totally missed quality of life. When I get cancer, THEN I can have surgery, then chemo and radiation, and finally I can take the toxic verzenio and aromatase inhibitors for the rest of my life. That sucks! And why would I want a life like that? Is it because I am old? At 65, I am being written off?

But I cannot escape the bias being thrown at me and I begin to think that maybe these other tests (the MBI and Contrast Enhanced Mammogram) might be acceptable options, allowing me to avoid surgery. By the time we leave, I have agreed to hold off on surgery and consult with my breast doctor again about these other options. *Maybe there is an answer besides surgery that is tolerable.* After leaving the surgeon's office, I go home and do some research. Both of the recommended alternative tests involve mammograms with injectable substances. One involves IV contrast and the other involves radioactive dye. I suspect that I might also react to these substances as I have started to react with these types of rashes and intense itching to strange and unknown conditions over the last several years – too many mosquito bites in a short time span, sunshine alone, and who knows what. Sometimes, the insanity rousing itching will last for up to six to eight weeks during which nothing provides relief. I am not sure I want to attempt any of these.

Back in the breast physician's office a few weeks later, I am met with the same attitude as the prior visit. Behind the scenes, there has been much discussion about my situation between the surgeon, genetics, and her with little agreement between parties about the best approach. Dr. Breast is reluctant to allow me to try the MBI. She mostly is stuck on having me do an MRI guided breast biopsy.

"They didn't find anything on the ultrasound," she declares, "so an MRI breast biopsy is necessary." *I am totally frustrated. What part of 'I am allergic to the dye' do you not understand?"*

"That is not true," I repeat to her several times, "They did see the area on the ultrasound, and it was not thought to be cancer." *Certainly, I am not the only one with this issue. There must be other methods of doing a biopsy.* But the doctor offers no other choices and I feel backed into a corner. I finally agree to schedule the MRI guided biopsy. But I feel like I have totally lost control of my life and am getting closer to refusing any interventions, of just going home and living my life until I die from whatever it is that is my fate. By the time I arrive home, I realize that I have just gone in a big circle. I am back where I started. I want relief from this craziness. I call to reschedule the mastectomies.

To top off the madness and add stress to the process, I discover that Medicare has denied payment for the visit to the surgeon because "the visit didn't indicate why it was medically necessary." I have only been on Medicare for six months and already this. I chose Original Medicare plus a top-of-the-line supplement because one supposedly doesn't need pre-authorization to see a specialist, and everything was supposed to be covered except a $226 deductible. Now I find out that they can willy nilly deny coverage for just about anything if they can deem it "medically not necessary." Where does it end? At the grave, I guess. I have begun to question all choices, but I am determined to follow the only path that seems to offer some freedom from constant contact with the medical system and their inflexible protocols. I think I am developing a panic disorder that is activated every time I see the inside of a clinic. I am hoping there is sunshine and happiness on the other side of this surgery.

CHAPTER 4

BILATERAL MASTECTOMIES WITH

GOLDIE LOCKS RECONSTRUCTION

Surgery is scheduled for Friday, March 31, 2023. My scheduled time to show up is 8:15 a.m. This tells me that I am not a first case, and it will be close to noon before surgery begins. Being a six-hour surgery, this concerns me that I have little time to recover afterward before the outpatient unit closes at 9 p.m. But there is not much I can do about it. I can only hope that everything will go smoothly.

My hubby and I arrive at the hospital around 7:30 a.m. The admission proceeds in an orderly and efficient manner. Then the wait begins. Around 9:45 a. m., I am wheeled to the pre-operative area. I send my hubby home to our daughter instead of sitting there anxiously waiting at the hospital. They will be sent texts periodically as the surgery progresses.

I am surprised when I am offered Celebrex, a nonsteroidal anti-inflammatory agent (NSAID) to be taken before surgery. I have been instructed not to take any NSAIDS for 48 hours after surgery because they can increase bleeding, so I find this perplexing. But I guess I am not to question such discrepancies. I do present my list of requests for the anesthesia side of things to the anesthesiologist. My one request is for Emend, a medication to prevent nausea.

"Sure," he says as he walks out the door. "Can you take a verbal order for that?" He directs his comment over his shoulder to the nurse.

"Yes," she responds but then discovers that she can't give this particular drug without a written order due to cost. This necessitates a call to the anesthesiologist again to request that he put the order in the electronic medical record. An hour later when it is time for me to go to the operating room, he still has not entered the order. My assigned nurse anesthetist, in order to keep things moving, pulls the drug from PYXIS (the drug dispensing unit in the OR) and comes to the pre-op area to administer it to me. I love nurse anesthetists. Afterall, this is what I have done for a living for 16 years now. They are that line of defense that is always at the bedside in the OR and providing for those small details that are so important to a great outcome for the patient. I drift off to sleep knowing that I am in good hands and will be well taken care of.

The first that I remember nine hours later is my daughter pushing Doane shortbread cookies towards my hand to eat. My brain is confused. I can't find the words to finish a sentence, so I sound like a rambling idiot. I am told later that I had an adamant conversation with the surgeon about the pain medication I wanted but I remember none of it and his response was, "You are not competent to make this decision right now." *No kidding*! Apparently, the nurses have also done all their required teaching on restrictions, drain care, and who to call if necessary but none of that is stored anywhere in my memory. I am thankful for my veterinarian daughter who has taken charge at this point. I have to ask her to repeat all of this information again at home. Within fifteen minutes of finally recovering my faculties, I am walking around the unit and headed home. I think they are eager to send this patient home. I also later wonder what in the world I all said to those around me for those two hours that are totally blanked out even though, I am told, I was awake and conversing.

Recovery at home continues smoothly. I am relieved to know that no cancer was found by the pathologist in the surgical specimens. The only task is to heal and get back to life. I take only two tramadol pain pills in the first two days. All I want to do is sleep after ingesting even a half of one, so I soon abandon that for alternating Tylenol and Duclofenac, another NSAID. This seems to control my pain well. By surgery day two, my daughter and I decide to take a peek at the result of the surgery. The Goldilocks reconstruction I chose uses the skin of the breasts to make a small mound on each side. I am pleased with the outcome – not too big, not too small, but just right without any extraneous materials or needing to take from other areas of the body. That is why they call it a Goldilocks. Goldilocks tried the big bed, the small bed, and finally, the medium size bed which was just right. I think I made the right choice. Well, maybe the right choice would have been to never have joined the Tapestry Study. Maybe not knowing one's genetic predisposition is the right choice. And for me, I think not knowing might have been the better choice from a mental health state, even if the intervention might potentially extend my life cancer free. I keep saying to others, "Think carefully about what you really want to know before joining a medical genetics study or have genetic testing done."

CHAPTER 5 $84,000 BILL.....

WHOA!

Though I heal physically with no complications, the financial end of things does not go nearly as well. The general surgeon's bill is one of the first to be processed. "Denied" is the verdict of Medicare for payment of the $10,600 general surgeon's portion of the bilateral mastectomies, the $3200 charge by pathology, and the over $4000 charge for my anesthesiologist and nurse anesthetist. It is denied because Medicare doesn't cover "routine care" or "preventative care." What a bunch of crock! How frustrating! Medicare does approve the $12,000 plastic surgery cost of the breast reconstruction as required by federal law. And Medicare, thankfully, approves the hospital facility usage portion amount of $42,000. So I am confused as to why they deny the doctor and other clinician's portions.

I immediately appeal Medicare's denial and I ask the hospital to check the correctness of the coding. I explain to them that the surgeon and I both contacted Medicare pre-operatively, attempting to determine how other surgeries such as mine had been handled by Medicare in the past and if a pre-authorization could be obtained. The standard answer from Medicare was, Original Medicare does not provide pre-authorizations. They only provide a determination after submission of the claim. I found that puzzling and a wee bit late once I am holding a gigantic, uncovered bill in hand.

I also explain to the billing department that I had made numerous contacts over the last two months with the clinic's accounting department in an attempt to resolve this issue so that I would not be doing what I am now doing – looking at a huge, uncovered bill. I had also asked the clinic for an estimate on the surgery amount so I would have some idea of what I was looking at if coverage was denied, but an estimate was never received. Finally, I explain that I was not presented with an "advanced beneficiary notice of non-coverage (ABN) which is required if the medical facility believes there is a possibility that a procedure will not be covered, leading me to believe that my surgery would be covered. For these reasons, I explain my position that I am not responsible for this bill. The clinic obviously is not impressed with my reasonings and chooses to ignore them. They come back saying the bill is coded properly and do not hesitate to post the approximately $12,000 denied by Medicare to my account. Medicare also comes back denying my appeal after a medical redetermination.

Every person I talk to in billing at the hospital and at Medicare gives me a different answer. Therefore, this uncovered portion of the procedure sits unmoving on my account over the course of several months. The hospital has no intention of working with me to resolve the charges. I ask my surgeon for a "letter of medical necessity" several times and even send him an example of what I need. He is very pleasant and says he will help in any way possible, but he never carries through with what I am requesting. I also ask him to include code R92.8 (Other abnormal and inconclusive findings on diagnostic imaging of breast) in the patient notes which is suggested to me by one of the billing specialists as an appropriate diagnostic code for my situation. This never happens either so coding cannot be changed, I am informed.

One day, I decide to make an in-person visit to the billing department at the clinic. I have a plan. I take along a typed document I have developed for billing to sign should they happen to accept my proposal. I begin by explaining all the reasons I do not legally owe them this bill. Then I make my offer.

"I will give you $2500 to cover the $12,000 that you say I owe you. This is more than Medicare would have paid you if they had approved the charges," I declare.

"We don't know how much Medicare would pay," is the first comeback.

"Oh, yes you do," I retort.

"Well, we can't do that," they insist. "The best we can do is give you a 10% discount."

I stare at the Accounts Department lady and leave her with my ultimatum. "Well, then you are not getting paid. You can turn it over to collections and I will offer them the $2500." I turn and walk away. So much for my trip downtown into this stressful crowd of people.

Two days later while working on the computer at home, the house phone rings, "We will accept your offer."

OK, I am taken off guard and I agree too quickly, "OK, how do you want me to pay?"

"If you could pay us with a debit card, that is what we would like."

What? My debit only allows $500 withdrawn per day. What is the point of insisting on a debit card rather than a credit card? We do finally agree on a credit card. But later, I realize that by doing this over the phone, I have not been able to have them sign my document stating that this payment is for the full remaining amount of any charges from March 31, the surgery day. And of course, I get a letter stating I might still owe $1800 for the pathology because the clinic is waiting for my supplemental insurance to respond to that bill. I hate to tell them my supplement has already denied it twice because Medicare denied it. There is no reason for them to approve or pay that $1800. I decide to wait until after the response to my next appeal to Medicare before I address this issue. At least the bill says zero for now. But before I get any response to my appeal, I am presented by Mayo with the $1800 bill. My supplemental insurance denied the claim as I expected they would. Another phone call to the billing department is needed as a result. And the same kind of conversation ensures as before. They reject my premise that my previous offer was to cover all of this.

"No that is not what the notes say," declares the unrelenting party. Finally in desperation, I offer them another $300 to cover the $1800 and get it removed from my account for now.

"Oh no. We can't do that." The standard answer of every account representative spews from her mouth.

"Give me a supervisor!" I demand, frustrated.

"I'm sorry," the supervisor says, "She didn't understand correctly. I will accept your $300 offer."

"I want a paper stating that this bill is totally covered by what I have paid you," is my definitive behest. "And if I win my appeal, I want my money back," is my final request. The clinic does send a final bill showing a zero balance a couple of weeks later.

CHAPTER 6

FINAL APPEALS AND CONCLUSION

By the first of November, I still have not received a response to my second level of appeal, the Medicare Reconsideration Decision. I know that I only have sixty days after their decision to make the next level of appeal to an administrative law judge. I finally call the number listed on my appeal paperwork. "Oh, we sent you a letter on September 29 informing you of an unfavorable decision." Great, not again! And I never received the decision letter; therefore, the lady promises to send me a duplicate copy. Another ten days pass before the promised ruling arrives. This only leaves me about two weeks to make my third appeal. I do notice under the section "Who is Responsible for this Bill?" an interesting statement, "The QIC finds that the provider is liable for the denied charges. The record does not support that the beneficiary was notified in advance with a properly executed Advance Beneficiary Notice that Medicare would likely deny payment for the service at issue. The beneficiary cannot be charged for these services." Wow!! This is exactly what I had tried to convey to Mayo when they initially posted the charges to my account, but they have chosen to totally ignore not only me, but Medicare as well.

By now, this has become a matter of principle rather than money. I am totally frustrated by a government agency that will not provide a pre-approval or denial of a surgery or procedure before the actual intervention has occurred but then refuses to pay for it because it is "routine" or "preventative" even though this is an accepted method of treatment for someone with the situation that I find myself in. Who made up these rules? Why would an insurance company not pay for an intervention that prevents future illness and saves tons of money in tests that are not needed any longer, medications that do not need to be bought, or chemotherapy and radiation that would be needed if cancer developed. I don't follow any of this logic. Our insurance system is totally messed up.

I debate as to whether I should proceed on to Appeal #3 which is to an Administrative Law Judge. Is it even worth my effort? The bill has been taken care of and according to the last ruling, I should be getting my money back. But there has been no movement by Mayo to that effect. What do I have to lose? I finally decide to proceed with the third level of appeal. The worst that can happen is that the appeal is denied for the third time.

My hearing date is originally set for Monday, December 18, 2023. I groan when I open the letter. Of the many dates they could have scheduled the hearing, it has been set for one of the only four days that I work in December. I send a fax detailing why I cannot be present that date and amazingly and without any further questions, the system changes it to December 19. It is not a hearing that I need to attend in person but a phone session. I am given a code to access the hearing at 10 a.m. CST. That seems simple enough and all I have to do is present my case as to why I think this surgery should be covered. I get a little nervous, though, when it is communicated to me that I am entitled to have legal representation. If I have to pay a lawyer too, then this is not worth it.

One day while I am working in the operating room in my role as a nurse anesthetist, my cell phone rings. I cannot take the call at that time and let it go to voicemail. The message, I find out later, is from Mayo's lawyers. I am shaken. "Whoa…? What is the meaning of this? Are they for me or against me? What could they possibly want?" In my callback, I learn that they have also received a summons to the court date but are declining to attend. However, they are offering me advice on how to proceed with my presentation. I am surprised that they are reaching out to me, but their counsel does reinforce that I am on the right path. I subsequently type out the points I want to cover.

The morning of the hearing, five minutes before the scheduled time, I dial the number and enter the code supplied in the mailing.

"The judge is not available at this time," the recording announces.

I call back in a couple of minutes. This time, after entering the passcode, I am instructed to enter the access code. Now I am confused. I was only given one code, so I re-enter it. "You have not entered the correct code," the machine says. Now I am frantic. I try again with the same result. Great!! Just great!! Looks like I am going to miss the hearing because I have no idea how to get in. But I try one more time, and this time I hit the # key as instructed "if you don't know the code" and it goes right through. I sigh and try to calm my now flustered appearance.

The judge is polite, friendly, and professional. "Show me why I should approve your claim," she begins. "Now is your opportunity to shine. Tell me what you see as different from the prior denials that I should be aware of."

"This was not a preventative surgery," I emphasize, "But one to address the abnormal findings of the MRI which is well documented in the notes of Dr. Breast on January 10, 2023. There would have been NO mastectomies if the MRI had been normal." When my declaration is met by silence, I ramble on, "I want to tell you my story…" and then I proceed to detail my personal story. "… bilateral mastectomies are standard medical treatment for high-risk individuals usually defined as persons having the BRCA1 and 2 genes of which I am," I finish. She continues to listen quietly, so I proceed on to explaining how it is cheaper to pay for a prophylactic bilateral mastectomy than to receive two to three years of cancer treatment. I highlight too that Medicare covers a number of preventative treatments (ie Flu shots, covid shots, bone marrow density tests, colonoscopies). I finish up with pointing out that many commercial insurance companies pay for prophylactic mastectomies, oophorectomies and hysterectomies for those having the BRCA 2 gene. In fact, my daughter's insurance, Blue Cross Blue Shield, is covering her recent surgery for an oophorectomy and a hysterectomy due to also being identified as carrying the same gene as me, the BRCA2.

"So were you ever given an estimate?" she at last questions.

"No, if you want to go there, I was not ever given an estimate even though I asked for one, nor was I given an Advanced Benefits Notice so I assumed that we were 'good to go' and I believed the clinic expected it to be covered."

"So have you been left with the $84,000 to pay personally?"

"No, my supplemental insurance paid part of it and Medicare paid the hospital side of the bill which makes no sense to me. Why would Medicare pay for the hospital part but not the doctor part? And I made an agreement with Mayo for the rest so it is all covered at this point."

"How much was your part that was billed to you?" she finishes.

"$12,000."

She has no more questions and offers no other thoughts. The hearing is closed. I have no idea if I have been successful. Waiting 60 – 90 days for the verdict is the next step.

I feel good about my presentation though and am convinced that this time my appeal will result in a successful ruling. Every day I peek in the mailbox hoping to see that envelope return-addressed from the Health and Human Services agency. Butterflies twit about my stomach the day in early February that it finally arrives. I can't wait to rip it open.

"After carefully considering the evidence presented in the record and at the hearing, I enter an UNFAVORABLE decision" begins the ten-page ruling from the judge. Disappointment and disbelief flood through me. Seriously…?? I methodically read through the document. After several readings, I gather that the Administrative Law Judge agrees that my record contains sufficient documentation to conclude that the services were not simply "routine" or "preventative" but does not contain sufficient evidence to conclude that they were "medically necessary" in that the record does not establish that a bilateral mastectomy was the standard next in line treatment option after MRI biopsy and surveillance. This seems to be based on the comments of the surgeon in the record that states that "molecular breast imaging" in addition to mammograms could be considered an alternative (to MRIs and mammograms). Of course, he does not mention that Molecular Breast Imaging also requires the use of IV dye. Besides that, I had gone back to Dr. Breast after my visit with the surgeon hoping that this avenue might be an option. But she was quick to say, "No, it confuses everything at this point. You really need to do the MRI guided biopsy first and then we can talk about it." Frustrated and trapped at that point would have been a huge understatement as no viable options were being presented. So just what does the judge think would have been the next "standard" line of treatment? Yep...It's do that allergy inducing MRI guided breast biopsy and then if negative, continue surveillance with potentially also allergy inducing MBI. Of course, if the biopsy is positive, continue with the same treatment as was done. This splitting of hairs is ridiculous. I would like to see these decision makers continue yearly with a test that causes them to break out in an itchy insanity inducing rash for six weeks.

But I am defeated at this point. Trying to force sanity from an insane system is impossible. I have no intention of pursuing the appeals to Medicare further. But I do send an email to the two medical lawyers who so graciously reached out to me to let them know the result. And I do contact the clinic accounts receivables department and again, for the third time, request the money that I paid be returned to me based on the Administrative Law Judge's second part of the ruling that the clinic is responsible for any non-covered costs because they "should have known" Medicare wouldn't cover this procedure. If Medicare won't tell someone a procedure is not covered before a claim is submitted, I don't know how the clinic is supposed to know either. But I tried to communicate to Mayo when they first started billing me that I never received an ABN or advanced notice that this would be an uncovered bill. However, they have continued to ignore this fact over the last year. Once I present the judge's final ruling, they raise no more objections and begin the process of returning the $2800 I paid them.

How The BRCA2 Gene Impacted My Life

Three and a half years have passed since I started on this journey. I reflect back on the that time and my decision to join the research study and mostly what I feel is regret. All knowing the results has done is cause anguish and a trip down a road that has led to decisions by both me and my daughter that we would have not otherwise made. It also caused the medical staff at the clinic to treat me in a totally different manner and with an urgency I did not feel was warranted. The sadness I feel at never having grandchildren is more profound than any worry about whether I might get breast cancer. Was the surgeon right that I would live just as long regardless of whether I had surgery or not? The attitude that living with cancer is just as good as living without it at age sixty-five I found a little disconcerting. But I certainly could have avoided all the recommended intensive monitoring along with its allergic reactions if I had never known I am BRCA2 positive. I am definitely happy with the freedom the surgery has given me to not need to be poked, stuck, and squished any more in my life. I am quite happy with the results of the surgery as well.

But I also learned a sad truth about our Medicare system. It is not designed to pay for people to seek preventative or routine care or to seek the lowest cost treatment option. Once you have cancer and are headed towards the grave, they will approve your claims and pay for your treatment and care but will make no effort to help you prevent it. This thought process and approach to what standards of care are appropriate is a little outdated in today's progressive society, I would think.

Mary Ellen Dreher

* 9 7 9 8 8 8 4 7 9 4 6 1 0 *